Champion's Vision

A Basketball Player's Before the Game Preparation Guide

David Smith

B180 Basketball, Inc.
P.O. Box 2406
Midland, MI 48641-2406
www.b180basketball.com
Phone: 1-800-957-1275

© 2017 by David Smith. All rights reserved.

No part of this book may be reproduced, stored in a retrieval system, or transmitted by any means without written permission from the author.

Published by B180 Basketball, Inc. 11/17/2017
ISBN: 978-1-7325361-1-1 (sc)
ISBN: 978-1-7325361-0-4 (e)

Library of Congress Control Number: 2017916939

Any people depicted in stock imagery are models, and such images are being used for illustrative purposes only.

Because of the dynamic nature of the Internet, any web addresses or links contained in this book may have changed since publication and may no longer be valid. The views expressed in this work are solely those of the author and do not necessarily reflect the views of the publisher, and the publisher hereby disclaims any responsibility for them.

Contents

Dedication iv
Acknowledgments v
Introduction 1
A Champion's Journey Begins with a Vision 2
Five Suggested Strategies to use as Preparation,
Days Before a Game.. 3
Chapters:
   1. The Pre-Game 13
   2. Half Time 18
   3. The Last 2 Minutes 25
   4. Overtime 31
   5. After the Game 37
   6. Practice Approach 41
   7. Strength & Fitness Training 45
   8. The Off-Season 50
   9. Pickup Games 54
   10. One on One 57
A Basketball Wish 60

Dedication

This book is dedicated to all the hardworking, passionate, determined, and goal oriented basketball players who stay in the gym countless hours in order to better their individual basketball skills, year in and year out.

Acknowledgments

I'd like to acknowledge the coaches that played a part in my development as a player, coach, and person. I can proudly say that as a basketball player in high school or college, each year that I played basketball, I was a part of a team that always had a winning end of season overall win/loss record. It all started with having great coaches and my willingness to sacrifice individual accomplishments for team success. It was all worth it. Mr. Jimmie Sanders, thank you for giving me the keys to the offense as the point guard at an early age in high school. I was a sophomore. You helped me to develop confidence, leadership, trust and commitment, the ability to run a team, and an understanding of the importance of giving back. Mr. Steve Schmidt, thank you for being there as a friend and coach; your commitment to developing positive and open communication with each of the players on the team is what makes you stand out as a coach. You are always there for any of your players. Your no excuses approach stood out, and it's what defines the players that have and will play for you. Mr. Dean Lockwood, thank you for helping me to develop discipline as a player and as a person. I admired your approach to daily practices, games, and the season as a whole. I'm glad and feel very fortunate that I had you as a coach. Mr. Bob Taylor, thank you for helping me to develop my skill set as a basketball player. Your keen understanding of what it takes to be the best player possible is admired. You truly are an asset to the basketball community.

Introduction

Throughout the history of basketball, players have had different ways of preparing before they actually played the game. As you may know, that preparation begins way before a couple of hours when the game is about to start. What happens when your mind is racing in every direction, you've prepared ahead of time, and you still need something to get you ready to play?

It begins with a vision, a certain state of mind. It begins with a plan. Leading up to the pre-game, there is a certain level of confidence that a player must have and maintain in order to get results.

This book and audio have been developed to help prepare basketball players as they journey before the game, and during the game. I hope that you have success along your journey and reach your goals & dreams in basketball.

Listen to the audiobook or read your favorite part of the paperback book before you play the game. If you have the chance at halftime, listen to or read it again. Do this before every game as part of your pre-game routine.

A Champion's Journey Begins with a Vision

*Team communication when on the floor together

What makes up the successful components of a basketball team?

When analyzing the coaches and players on a basketball team, it's comparable to a boxer. The point guard is the head and mind of the boxer. The shooting guard is an arm of the boxer. The wing is an arm of the boxer. The four man is a leg of the boxer. The five man is a leg of the boxer. The coaches are the knowledge, discipline, heart, and determination of the boxer. The bench players are the motivation of the boxer. Everyone is needed.

Five Suggested Strategies to use as Preparation, Days Before a Game

- Think Positive Thoughts
- Eat Smart
- Watch Film
- Review and Rest
- Complete Non-Game Related Tasks Early

Think Positive Thoughts

The thought process is the most important part of an individual's preparation for a basketball game. Having a clear picture in your mind of yourself being successful begins to bring what you see in your mind into reality. There is no such thing as a shooting or game slump if you can master the art of thinking positive. Draw on paper and outline in your mind a mental map of everything you need to do to perform at a high level on game day. Visualize yourself doing positive things before and during the game.

There was a time in practice as a college basketball player, that I was physically drained.

We had run, did drill after drill, and scrimmaged. We had one more scrimmage left. In order for me to stay focused and perform at a high level, I started to think and say positive words of encouragement to myself. I felt this played an important part in me having the energy to continue practicing.

As a former head basketball coach, I got the chance to see the actual power of thinking positive during preparation before game day. I had a player that went through a pre-game warm-up and the actual game in his mind after studying the scouting report. He'd picture the opposing player that he had to guard. He'd see himself playing stellar defense, stealing the ball from the player. Then dribbling down court and scoring the basketball while getting fouled. This is positive thinking!

The way you think controls a lot of things that lead up to game day. If you have negative actions that cloud your thoughts, try channeling those negative things out through strength training, watching film, laughing, being around positive people, and working out on the basketball court. Maintain a tunnel vision of positive thinking.

Eat Smart

What you put in your body determines a lot about your ability to maintain a high-level performance during the game. Said a little different, eating and loading up with sugar and other unhealthy options before the basketball game takes away how long you are able to be dominant

in an actual game. Be a smart and healthy consumer of food before games. In that case, why not be health conscious when choosing food all of the time? You'll see changes in a lot of areas in your health and way of living. Know what you are putting in your body at all times. Yes, this means watching what medications you use as well. Seek out advice of alternative, healthier and safer options before completely choosing a medication.

As a high school freshman basketball player, I remember when I'd eat two quarter pounders, a large fry, and drink a coke about two and a half hours before playing in a basketball game. Was this really a healthy and smart choice? Though I thought I was performing at an elite level during the game, in hindsight, I wasn't even close. Over the years, I've become a healthier consumer of food. I'm a vegetarian now, well, almost a vegetarian. I'm a pescetarian because I do eat most kinds of fish, but no other type of meat. I gradually changed my eating habits over the years. The in-game results as well as how I felt was a sign that I was making better eating choices. I'm not suggesting that you become a vegetarian. I'm suggesting that you listen to your trainer or dietitian when it comes to eating smart and maintaining a healthy diet that prepares you to perform at the highest level during practice and games.

When I coached, I used the following after game meal option for away games. It was called "sub, sub, pizza." To explain, for an away game, number one we'd have healthy fruit and snacks before the game. After the game, we'd have a healthy sub sandwich option with a low-fat side item, as well as a healthy drink option. We'd eat that way two away games in a row, and then we'd get pizza for the after game meal for the third away game. This isn't by any means the healthiest eating choice for a team, but I believed that it helped the players become more aware of what they were putting into their bodies. We would also eat fruit during halftime of our games.

Watch Film

When you begin to watch game film, you become a student of the game. Whether on offense or defense, your eyes begin to open as you become aware of the opportunities available on a typical possession. An overall understanding of your own strengths and weaknesses can be seen, corrected, and mastered. Weaknesses can now become strengths of yours if they are acknowledged, acted upon, and developed with practice. When preparing days before a basketball game, you should watch and study your opponent's team offensive and defensive tendencies. Also, analyzing offensive and defensive tendencies of the individual opponent you will be matched up against should be done several times. By the time of the actual game day, you should know your opponent's strengths and weaknesses; just as good as you know yours. When watching film, for example, paying attention to where your opponent catches the ball once in-bounded, and which way the individual typically turns before dribbling or passing the ball while being pressed full court is an example of how you can gain a competitive advantage when your team decides to press full court. You hear the great ones discuss the importance of watching and breaking down film all of the time. Watching film improves your basketball IQ, as well as your approach to in-game team and individual strategies to use on your opponent.

As a basketball player, I didn't truly realize the importance of watching film until around my junior year in high school. I'd try to gain a competitive advantage by taking away the strength of my individual opponent and by forcing him to use his weakness. I'd try to listen to the name of a particular offensive play. For example, if the name of the play on the scouting report and on film was called "Box 2." When "Box 2" is called, the two-guard goes off a series of screens for the catch and shot. I would attempt to anticipate the pass or disrupt the ball handler based on how they executed the play on the film that I watched.

Review and Rest

When it's time to review, it includes many aspects. Review includes examining team practice goals, individual practice goals, strength & conditioning goals, individual & team season goals, opponent scouting reports, Individual & team game strategies for the opponent, nutrition goals & plans, and your overall daily & weekly tasks. Reviewing everything keeps you accountable. You are able to track your progress towards individual and team goals. You are also able to mentally prepare for and clear up any misunderstandings as it relates to the game strategies that are planned for your opponent.

Resting involves a time for you to recover from the overuse of your mind and your physical body. A time set aside to rest should happen daily. In order for you to play and perform at an elite level, your mind and body need time daily to rest and recover. You are probably saying, what should I do when I rest? Some of the things to consider when resting are sleeping, listening to music, laughing, reading, meditating, getting a massage, or any non-physical labor activity that is healthy and safe for you. Try as much as possible to stay off of your feet. Don't stand for long periods of time. Remember you've been running, jumping, sliding, and strength training with your legs at an extreme level. They need rest.

As a coach, I gave each player a scouting report that outlined our opponent's team strengths and weaknesses. The scouting report also included a breakdown of each individual player on our opponent's team. It outlined their strengths and weaknesses too. What I found to be true as a result of doing this was that the players on our team that read and studied the scouting report on their own, outside of the team meetings had better in-game performances against that particular team.

As a player, I wanted to always be the smartest person on the court. I would watch game film and study the scouting reports on my own time. This had a great impact on my defensive performance during games. I also became very knowledgeable of quickly analyzing a basketball player to find out his or her basketball strengths and weaknesses.

Review and rest plays an important part in your long-term season success. You don't want to burn out prior to the season being over. Listen carefully to your coaches' game and practice plans. Likewise, listen to your trainers and dietitian. Follow the plan that's outlined for you. Take advantage of every opportunity to review and rest days before the actual game.

Complete Non-Game Related Tasks Early

Getting non-game related task done early relieves stress and anxiety. Procrastination is not an option. Non-game related tasks can include a multitude of tasks or events that an individual has throughout their daily life. Examples are course homework, projects, family events, personal relationship events, meetings and presentations, volunteer opportunities, running a business or working a job. When a plan of action is not in place to complete these events or tasks, the individual loses focus from the upcoming game plan. Their time, energy, and thoughts are divided among all of the tasks or events that need to be completed, as well as the upcoming basketball game. By being able to plan to complete events or tasks earlier in the day or the week, the player will be able to clear his mind, have available time to rest, and do other game-related tasks. Start planning two to four weeks in advance for events and tasks that you have the ability to schedule early.

As a coach, I included study hall as part of practice on a weekly basis. This gave each player added time to complete stressful assignments as well as seek out help. The players would receive a season-long completed schedule of every practice we had planned too. This aided them in their scheduling of events and tasks that were important to them.

As a college basketball player, I would study during my down times. I also would try to plan my important non-basketball tasks and events in the morning or afternoon. I am a morning person, so this worked best for me. When it came to scheduling group meetings or doctor appointments, I made sure that I had a clear understanding of how long each appointment took, and what other tasks or events I had remaining to schedule. The most important tasks and events were scheduled first.

Chapter 1

Chapter 1
The Pre-Game

The pre-game is a time when you have to maintain mental focus. Clearly listen and understand your team's game plan. By this time, you should know your opponent scouting report, as well as your individual opponent's strengths and weaknesses. A plan of attack should be visualized as well as written out on how you plan to deliver the best in-game performance possible.

It's ok to do a very light strength-training workout before the game. It relieves stress and tension. Make sure it's finished by at least an hour and a half before game tips off. When you are warming up on the court, try to make a shot from every spot on the floor that you would take in the game. It's a must. Warming up at game speed will have you better prepared for the actual tip off and start of the game than just going through the motions. Make sure every thought you have is always a positive one. Don't waste time talking or interacting with your opponent until after the game ends.

I remember the first time I lifted weights before a game. I thought initially that it was going to throw off my shot. I did a very light workout. Then I wanted to be alone, so I sat in the locker room and just began to stare at the scouting report. I wasn't even listening to music. I didn't know why I was doing this. I began to visualize myself stealing the ball in the open court from the offensive player. I smiled to myself. After about twenty minutes or so, other players began to come into the locker room. Then the coaches came in. We went over the scouting report as a team, then went out to warm up. Throughout the warm-up, I just had this feeling that I was going to have a good game. I kept picturing myself doing things that were good. I did have a good game. I know that my initial thoughts about me being successful and actually seeing it in my own mind played a part in my in-game success.

What follows are some positive thought suggestions for The Pre-Game:

Say this to yourself five (5) times

   I'm having a good game today.
   I'm having a good game today.
   I'm having a good game today.
   I'm having a good game today.
   I'm having a good game today.

   All of my shots are going in.
   All of my shots are going in.
   All of my shots are going in.
   All of my shots are going in.
   All of my shots are going in.

I'm the best player on the court.
I'm the best player on the court.
I'm the best player on the court.
I'm the best player on the court.
I'm the best player on the court.

I broke their press and scored.
I broke their press and scored.
I broke their press and scored.
I broke their press and scored.
I broke their press and scored.

I'm making my free throws today.
I'm making my free throws today.
I'm making my free throws today.
I'm making my free throws today.
I'm making my free throws today.

I'm dropping 32 points with ease today.
I'm dropping 32 points with ease today.
I'm dropping 32 points with ease today.
I'm dropping 32 points with ease today.
I'm dropping 32 points with ease today.

Champion's Vision Tips #1

1. Keep your thoughts focused on positive things. Avoid distractions and negative people or situations before a big game or rival game.

2. Time management is important. Arrive at the facility on game day at least an hour earlier than what's required by your coaches or organization.

3. When extreme events occur such as a bench clearing brawl or other events and situations that are out of your control, don't get involved. Go to the locker room or seek shelter away from the situation for your safety. Be a leader during this time.

4. Don't talk with your spouse or significant other before, at halftime, or during the basketball game if you've been arguing with the person. Keep your mind clear of negative thoughts and focus on positive things. If you can't think of anything that's positive, reflect on a positive childhood event that got you to where you are today in the sport that you love.

5. Block out parents, family, and friends that are trying to talk to you during the game. You already have gotten advice before the game from them. Remind them of this well before the actual game starts. For maximum results, this must be done.

Chapter 2

Chapter 2
Half Time

Halftime is a time to evaluate what's working or not with your initial plan of action.

Discard and burn from your memory anything that did not go well for you in the first half. Listen carefully to your team's adjustments and in-game strategies for the next half. Adjust your individual performance level to focus and capitalize on the things that you are doing well.

Strive to improve on doing the basic things (such as make smart passes, make the open shot, box out smart, rebound, make layups, make your free throws, and play smart defense) at a great level in the next half. As it relates to your individual opponents, find out what worked best when you made them use a weakness of theirs. Continue to force your opponent to use a weakness that they are very bad at doing in the game. An example of this would be if your opponent is bad at making left-hand layups, force them into having no choice but to attempt a left-hand layup.

Make sure that you stretch out again then warm up at game speed. Try to make a shot from every spot on the court that you would in the game. Don't waste time talking or joking with your opponent until the game ends. Make sure that every thought you have is a positive thought going into the next half.

I remember in high school; it was our district finals basketball game. We were down by nineteen points at the half. My teammates' mood was that of uncertainty. The other captains and I began to say positive things to each of the teammates, as well as to each other. Coach then came into the locker room, and we all got quiet. I thought for sure that we were going to get a yelling that we haven't heard before. To my surprise, coach just simply grabbed a piece of chalk and wrote one single word on the board. He wrote the word "Heart." Then he walked away. That was all I needed to see. I began to picture myself working out as a little boy. I saw in my mind all of the work that I had put in over the summers to get better. I began to analyze my opponent. I knew that my opponent hadn't put in the amount of work in basketball as I did up to that point. I felt a lack of achievement because our opponent was up by nineteen points in the district finals at halftime. From that point, I knew that I had to bring it. In the next half, I forced the person that I was guarding to do the things that they were not good at and that they didn't do well in the first half. I forced the tempo. I pictured myself as an unstoppable playmaking force. My teammates followed. We came back and won that game. This game taught me the importance of motivation, as well as remembering to reward yourself for all of the sweat, time, and work that you put into basketball over the summer months. From that point on, I began to analyze the person that I was guarding even more. I paid attention to what was really working at halftime, and what could be adjusted as it relates to one-on-one match-ups.

What follows are some positive thought suggestions for Halftime:

Say this to yourself five (5) times

   I'm making the last second shot.
   I'm making the last second shot.
   I'm making the last second shot.
   I'm making the last second shot.
   I'm making the last second shot.

   I'm dropping dimes today.
   I'm dropping dimes today.
   I'm dropping dimes today.
   I'm dropping dimes today.
   I'm dropping dimes today.

   I've got lock-down defense today.
   I've got lock-down defense today.
   I've got lock-down defense today.
   I've got lock-down defense today.
   I've got lock-down defense today.

   I'm a beast on the boards today.
   I'm a beast on the boards today.

I'm a beast on the boards today.
I'm a beast on the boards today.
I'm a beast on the boards today.

Nobody can stop my inside game today.
Nobody can stop my inside game today.
Nobody can stop my inside game today.
Nobody can stop my inside game today.
Nobody can stop my inside game today.

Nobody can stop me from scoring today.
Nobody can stop me from scoring today.
Nobody can stop me from scoring today.
Nobody can stop me from scoring today.
Nobody can stop me from scoring today.

Nobody can stop my perimeter game today.
Nobody can stop my perimeter game today.
Nobody can stop my perimeter game today.
Nobody can stop my perimeter game today.
Nobody can stop my perimeter game today.

I'm winning the game for my team today.
I'm winning the game for my team today.
I'm winning the game for my team today.
I'm winning the game for my team today.
I'm winning the game for my team today.

I see the swish of the net as the ball goes in.
I see the swish of the net as the ball goes in.
I see the swish of the net as the ball goes in.

I see the swish of the net as the ball goes in.
I see the swish of the net as the ball goes in.

My next shot is going in.
My next shot is going in.
My next shot is going in.
My next shot is going in.
My next shot is going in.

Champion's Vision Tips #2

1. Have discussions and compliment teammates on the positive things they did during the game. Never blame teammates for mistakes.

2. Motivate yourself and your teammates at halftime of the game. Get everyone involved and committed to reaching the team goals for the second half of the game.

3. Be professional and courteous when being interviewed before, during, or after a basketball game. You are not only representing your team; you represent the people you care about the most, and your family.

4. Overcome poor first half performances by making plays on defense, free throws, smart passes, and layups. Think positive.

5. If you didn't play much or at all in the first half, motivate yourself by analyzing and watching the individuals on the other team that you would defend if you were in the game. Watch the tendencies of your opponent's offense and defense. When you are put into the game, you will have success. Be a positive and supportive team member, regardless of if you get into the game.

Chapter 3

Chapter 3
The Last 2 Minutes

This is the time when the great and elite players deliver memorable in-game performances. During this time period, a person must have laser focus. There is extreme harmony that's developed by the individual player and the flow of the game. This is passed on by the individual player to their teammates and coaches. Everything must result in something positive happening for your team. On offense, you are driving to the basket to make the layup, get fouled, and make your free throws or make a smart pass that leads to a made layup. This is a must. If you take a jump shot, it has to go in.

Extreme confidence must be had during this time. Visualizing what you've been doing well in the game up to this point as well as visualizing yourself making your favorite shot is an image that must be constantly pictured your mind and thoughts. Making the game-winning pass can be visualized as well.

Listen to what your opponent's coaches and players are saying as far as their in-game strategy goes. Being aware of the situation will help you make the smart play at the right time. Never believe that your team is out of a contest or will lose the game. Always think "one more." That's one more basket, and one more defensive stop will bring your team closer to a win. Make sure every thought is a positive one during the last two minutes of the game.

As a coach, we had a drill called the "last two minutes." The players would do a timed sprint down and back the full length of the basketball court two times. They then would select one person to make two free throws in a row. If they missed, we would have to do the timed sprints again. Then another player would be selected to make free throws. This helped our team to develop mental toughness at the most important times during basketball games. There was one particular game that stood out. We were playing a conference opponent. They were up eight points with a little over two minutes to play in the game. It was in a timeout that I reminded our players about what kind of mentality we have to have in the last two minutes of a game. Coming out of the timeout, the group for us that was on the floor had unwavering focus. They had a championship caliber communication level on defense and offense that I wish I could have bottled up and used again and again. Our opponent only scored two points I believe in those last two minutes, and we came back and won the game.

What follows are some positive thought suggestions for the Last 2 Minutes of the Game:

Say this to yourself five (5) times

I'm making all of the right plays.
I'm making all of the right plays.
I'm making all of the right plays.
I'm making all of the right plays.
I'm making all of the right plays.

I'm going to get a steal and a score after a timeout.
I'm going to get a steal and a score after a timeout.
I'm going to get a steal and a score after a timeout.
I'm going to get a steal and a score after a timeout.
I'm going to get a steal and a score after a timeout.

I don't feel any pressure.
I don't feel any pressure.
I don't feel any pressure.
I don't feel any pressure.
I don't feel any pressure.

I do my best in situations like this.
I do my best in situations like this.
I do my best in situations like this.
I do my best in situations like this.
I do my best in situations like this.

I'm winning this game for someone special.
I'm winning this game for someone special.
I'm winning this game for someone special.
I'm winning this game for someone special.
I'm winning this game for someone special.

I'm the best player.

I'm the best player.
I'm the best player.
I'm the best player.
I'm the best player.

Nobody can guard me.
Nobody can guard me.
Nobody can guard me.
Nobody can guard me.
Nobody can guard me.

Champion's Vision Tips #3

1. When taking the last shot, try to get to and shoot the basketball from your favorite spot on the court.

2. Make all of your free throws during the last minutes of a basketball game.

3. Block the referees out of the game by not responding to any calls that they make for or against your team. Let them do their job. Anticipate questionable calls by keeping your team ahead in the game score by at least a 10-point margin. This is a must for away contests.

4. Analyze both your teammates and your opponent based on their strengths and weaknesses. Visualize and create the next two to three plays in your mind. Then perform the plays in the real game.

5. Handle wins by being humble, and handle defeats with pride. Keep the focus on your long-term goals.

Chapter 4

Chapter 4
Overtime

It's a win at all cost. Leave your mark! This is a game when you've truly met your match on a particular day. The game strategies are even. What separates the winner of this game will be before game preparation, mental toughness and focus, or pure basketball luck. To prepare for this moment, you have to start thinking about what you've done in practice. Before leaving the gym after practice, did you do the "show stopper countdown?" Well, if you are not familiar with it, let me explain. It's you with the ball and there are five seconds left on the clock. Start counting down and before you count to zero, shoot the basketball and make it. Pure Show Stopper! Don't leave the gym until you make the shot at game speed.

In overtime, your mental focus has to be flawless. You have to be tuned in to the next two or three plays down court before they happen. Know your team's game plan going into overtime, as well as your opponents. Listen to what your coaches are saying about their strategy for overtime. Listen to what your opponent says during this time as it relates to game strategy very carefully. Whether playing defense or offense, you have to incorporate the last two minutes strategy from the start. Make every possession a positive outcome. The words you speak and the thoughts you have in your mind must be positive. Do the simple things in a great way.

A game that stood out to me was one that I played in as a player. It was a regional championship game. It went to double overtime. We had traded blow for blow with our opponent. It was an even draw for the entire game. It was pure coaching and pure smart basketball players playing on the court on both sides. After the score ended in a tie in regulation and the first overtime, we began to see on both sides a more assertive attempt to try and take charge of the game. Each team traded basket for basket. I orchestrated everything from the point guard position the entire game. With about a little less than a minute left in the double overtime game, I fouled out. I think we were up at the time. As I walked to the bench, I could see the opposing team celebrating as if they had won the game already. There was complete silence from the players on our team that was on the court. I couldn't stand to watch the remainder of the game. I was so sick to my stomach. However, as the time counted down, I began to feel ok with our chances. We were still up by one point with about twenty seconds to go. The opposing team had the ball. They came down, passed it around to the best player on the opposing team, and he missed. We didn't get the rebound. Our opponent ended up getting the rebound and passing it out to another player on their team. At this point, there were about seven seconds left in the game. Without hesitation, he shoots a three-pointer, and it goes in. As we scrambled to take the ball out, time expired. We lost the game. I couldn't believe it. Our team got beat by a shot that I had practiced day after day with devotion. Could I have made a difference if I was still on the court? Yes. I learned a lot from this game. I knew that I had to hold myself more accountable as a leader. I learned that you can't sit on the sideline in the most important times if you are the captain. From that point on, I began to strive to make sure I was on the court at the most important time in the game. I also want the ball at that time of the game to make it happen. This experience carried over to real the world and living a certain way of life for me as well.

What follows are some positive thought suggestions for overtime.

Say this to yourself five (5) times

   I'm going to get an And 1.
   I'm going to get an And 1.
   I'm going to get an And 1.
   I'm going to get an And 1.
   I'm going to get an And 1.

   I'm scoring from my favorite spot next time down court.
   I'm scoring from my favorite spot next time down court.
   I'm scoring from my favorite spot next time down court.

I'm scoring from my favorite spot next time down court.
I'm scoring from my favorite spot next time down court.

My next 3 pointer is going in.
My next 3 pointer is going in.
My next 3 pointer is going in.
My next 3 pointer is going in.
My next 3 pointer is going in.

My next pass will lead to a score.
My next pass will lead to a score.
My next pass will lead to a score.
My next pass will lead to a score.
My next pass will lead to a score.

I'm taking a charge.
I'm taking a charge.
 I'm taking a charge.
I'm taking a charge.
I'm taking a charge.

The referee's call does not matter
The referee's call does not matter
The referee's call does not matter
The referee's call does not matter
The referee's call does not matter

We will win the game.
We will win the game.
We will win the game.
We will win the game.

We will win the game.

Champion's Vision Tips #4

1. Make hustle plays, smart passes, free throws, and layups in overtime.

2. Move your feet and play smarter on offense and defense when you are playing with only one foul left to give. Talk aloud more to your teammates on defense.

3. Visualize the basketball already going in the basket before you even shoot the ball when taking the last shot.

4. Block out the crowd and negative things by focusing on your opponents offensive and defensive strategies. Visualize yourself making positive plays during the game.

5. After fouling out of a game, encourage your teammates in a positive way. Be a leader.

Chapter 5

Chapter 5
After the Game

Whether you win or lose after the game, shake hands with your opponent. The way you handle this step defines your character as a person. Never let one game get you too overjoyed or too down. There is more to be done to reach your team and individual goals. Well, you may ask, what if it's the championship game and your team won it all? I say, enjoy the moment, but get back to work because every team and every player are now working harder to get what you have. Enjoying what you have accomplished when a regular season game is over tends to be much different than when you are playing a tournament or championship game. The stakes are higher during tournament and championship time. If it's not the championship game that your team has just played for, then victories or defeats shouldn't be in the attention spotlight that long.

After the game is a time to meet with teammates and coaches first. Briefly discuss what went well in the game and what needs more work. Once that meeting is complete, you can see friends and family. Remember to rest and eat healthy during this time.

As a high school freshman basketball player, my team made it to the state semi-final game. Our team lost the state semi-final game to the eventual state champions. I had vowed to myself to make it to the state championship game and win it all before I graduated high school. That didn't happen. I remember our team's tone of behavior after that game. It was mixed. Part of the team was enjoying the moment because it was a great accomplishment for our school and community. The other members of the team had a look on their face of wanting to start preparing for next season that night. This experience taught me to always remember your long range goals and don't let a setback deter you from the original plan. Keep everyone on the same page as it relates to team long-term goals. As far as individual goals go, hold yourself accountable and find someone you trust that can help you hold yourself accountable. Always try to raise the bar. That's what keeps a person motivated and striving to be the best they can be.

After playing a game, it's important to gather your thoughts and care for any injuries that you have. Stay far away from negative people and influences. When it's time for the next game, you should have mentally put the previous contest that you played in behind you. Everything that you think about has to still be positive. Don't dwell on mistakes. Instead, try perfecting the areas that you struggled with in the game at practice. Watch film too.

Champion's Vision Tips #5

1. Shake your opponent's hand regardless of the outcome of the game.

2. If you didn't play in the game, analyze your strengths and weaknesses in basketball. In the next practice, try to dominate using your strengths. Work on improving your weaknesses in practice too. Stay thinking positive.

3. Celebrate after a win, knowing that you have more work to do. Expect to be successful. Acknowledge and thank your opponent for the good competition.

4. Do not get too depressed or down after a loss. Get back to work on your goals. Start thinking positive thoughts about the next basketball game.

5. Be aware of your emotions when getting interviewed after a game. Take a moment to think before you respond to a question.

Chapter 6

Chapter 6
Practice Approach

The approach that should be taken to practice is that of a game. Everything that you would do before and during an actual game should be done in practice. Repetition after repetition is the key. Your coaches will outline and discuss specific drills with you and the team during this time. Listen carefully first, then perform the drills at game speed every time. Mistakes will happen. Learn quickly from the mistakes. If you are able to perform in practice at a high level, you'll begin to set yourself up for success in the actual game. When you are competing in drills and scrimmages, choose to guard the best or one of the better teammates on your team. This will force you to raise your level of play. Likewise, if you are participating and performing at a very high level in practices, then the teammate that you are going up against will be forced to raise their level of play as well. This makes you and your team more prepared for actual games. Practices will and must get physical at times. Don't whine complain, or pout. Just get better. If you are able to play through a good, fun, and competitive practice without complaining or talking negative, it will raise your basketball game to another level.

As a coach, I saw the effects of how not complaining and always staying positive does good things for a team. We were in practice, and we had a tough conference game coming up that week. The practices were very physical. It was clean tough competition. In our scrimmages, we had a rule that there were no fouls and no dribbles allowed. They went full court during the scrimmages too. Now the opponent we played that particular week was an even match for us. They were talented but undisciplined at times. Since our players took to learning teamwork and staying positive in a good way during our practices leading up to the game, we were able to handle all of the negative things that went on in that game in a positive and disciplined way. Our team had developed mental toughness because of this experience.

Champion's Vision Tips #6

1. Work on and develop the skills and areas you know that you are weak in during practice.

2. Have a clear understanding of all of your team's offensive and defensive plays. Know all five positions.

3. Dominate during scrimmages on the defensive end by getting one-on-one stops and causing turnovers. Dominate on offense using a weakness that you have. Improve on your strengths too.

4. Strive to be first during drills and timed conditioning runs.

5. Strive to compete against and beat the better players on the team at every practice.

Chapter 7

Chapter 7
Strength & Fitness Training

A plan of action should be written out for your strength & fitness training goals. Create a plan for 1) before the season, 2) in-season, 3) after-season, and 4) the off-season. Your training programs should include more than just strength & agility training workouts. It should include a proper dieting plan, flexibility or proper stretching workouts, and exercises to maintain long term health. Remember you only got one body. So plan to develop and nurture it for the present and future years. When your playing days are done, you'll still want to be able to have good all around health and flexibility. A description of strength & fitness training plans by season follows.

*Note - The descriptions and suggestions that follow are the author's views. Check with your trainer if needed.

<u>Strength & Fitness Training Plans</u>

Before the Season:

This plan should focus on preparing your body for the long season and playoffs. Conditioning, as well as core strength, should be a focus. Strength training should be done. The use of heavy weights while strength-training during this time period should not be done. Before the season, training plans should last one to one and a half months.

In-Season:

The plan should focus on maintaining strength, flexibility, and proper dieting. During the long season, don't overlook the importance of stretching and eating healthy. Strength training during this time should be done using light weight and more repetitions. In-season plans should last five to six months.

After-Season:

The plan should focus on flexibility, core strength, and recovery exercises. The season just ended. Your body needs rest and recovery. You still want to maintain a level of physical activity, but rest, recovery, and flexibility are the primary focus and should be adhered to strategically. If there is strength training present, use light weights when lifting. After-season training plans should last one and a half months to two months.

Off-Season:

The plan should focus on strength, agility, core strength, proper dieting, and flexibility.

During this time, you are training for growth in every area: basketball skills, physically and mentally. The workouts should be intense but not overboard. Maintain a good diet during this time. Off-season training programs should last two to three months.

As a basketball player, I tried to maintain a good strength-training plan as well as made sure that I had time to devote to basketball skill workouts on the court. This was done outside of what my coaches had planned for the team. The basketball skill workouts were more intense during the off-season. The toughest problem you may come up against is managing your time for doing both. With the help of your trainer, write out a plan of action for both strength & fitness training and basketball skill workouts. Make eighty percent of the workouts. This will set you up for growth and success during the season.

Champion's Vision Tips #7

1. When strength training, use proper form and techniques. Lifting too much weight at one time can cause injuries if not done correctly.

2. Wear t-shirts that cover your biceps to the weight room. This will make the workout go faster. It eliminates the time spent looking in the mirror at yourself.

3. Stretch after lifting weights.

4. Find a partner to strength and fitness train with. They will keep you accountable for showing up.

5. Joke sparingly during workouts. It's ok to joke when the workout session is over.

Chapter 8

Chapter 8
The Off-Season

The time to get better is the off-season. A clear thought out plan of specific areas that you want to improve on the most should be done. Talk with your coaches, trainers, and dietitian to come up with a plan. Also, review your goals from the season that just ended. Analyze what went well and what needs to be improved. During the off-season, there is a tendency to get easily distracted. There possibly will be so much going on in your daily life that you can't find enough time to get a good workout done. To make sure that you fit your off-season workouts in your schedule, it's suggested to use the 5am-8am time block to workout. Why five o'clock in the morning? Because it's one of the first things that you will do on a particular day and it holds you accountable to get rest at night. Discipline yourself to wake up and be on time to the gym or strength & fitness training facility. If you finish before eight o'clock in the morning, it's fine.

Just make sure that you complete your entire scheduled workout for that particular day. The off-season strength workouts should be done with a partner. This partner will also be able to motivate you and hold you accountable.

As a coach, I coached a player that stayed committed to his off-season workout program. He played his first year as a true freshman at a listed height of 6'5 and 185 pounds. He, unfortunately, injured himself and had to sit out the entire next season. When he came back the following season, his hard work and dedication to strength training and basketball skill training had paid off. He had grown taller to be 6'6 and now weighed 215 pounds of solid muscle. He had a great season. He truly earned and deserved everything that he accomplished. This included a First Team All-Conference selection. Stay committed to your off-season plan. You will be happy that you did when it's time for the season to begin.

Champion's Vision Tips #8

1. In order to maintain consistency of summer workouts and growth, plan vacations strategically.

2. Spend more time working on reaching your personal goals. Attend less parties given by friends, family, or associates.

3. Spend time with your spouse or significant other often during the off-season.

4. Spend time with your family and friends during the off-season. Limit the number of parties you attend.

5. Watch film, read books and improve yourself as a person. Be a student of the game and a lifelong learner.

Chapter 9

Chapter 9
Pickup Games

Pickup games can be a good time to work on the weak areas of your game. That is if you consistently play competitively at a high level and game speed. If you are just going to coast or just go through the motions, don't play at all. You will see that your opponent won't show any mercy on you and will try to bring their best. Instead, be dominant and develop your weaknesses. You have to decide if playing in pickup games are really worth it, given the After Season and Off-Season plans that you have made. Prioritize your scheduled plans. After-Season and Off-Season workouts should be done before you play in a pickup game. When playing pickup games, always guard the best player on the opposing team. This will help you as you strive to develop your weaknesses. Follow the same procedures that you would follow in practice or game, as far as stretching and warming up goes.

As a player, I tried to play pick-up basketball games a lot. I developed the weak areas of my game by using the pick-up games as a practice. I always strive to be the smartest player on the basketball court and the most vocal. The verbal exchanges that I had were done in a positive and motivating way for me to push myself to another level. I quickly strive to develop an understanding of the strengths and weaknesses of the people that were on my team, as well as the people that we were going up against. This should be something that's mastered. When I played pick-up ball during the off-seasons while I was still in college, my main goal was to strictly be dominant using only a weakness I had at the time.

Overall, find a balance between your workouts and the amount of pick-up ball you will play. It's beneficial.

Champion's Vision Tips #9

1. When playing pick-up games, don't play on a team that has all of the best players in the gym on it. Instead, go against them and get better.

2. Play and learn different basketball positions during pick-up games.

3. Learn to be dominant while giving or receiving trash talk. Don't lose your focus. Stay thinking positive. Control your emotions, regardless of the situation or what was said. Let your on-court performance speak for you.

4. Go full speed when playing in pick-up games.

5. Guard the best players when playing in pick-up games.

Chapter 10

Chapter 10
One on One

If there was a magic potion that creates a great basketball player, then this is it. You must be able to create your own shot from any area on the court against any style of defender. You also must be able to defend and shut down any type of offensive player. Challenging the best players on your team to play one-on-one helps you become better. Work on your weaknesses as well as your strengths when playing. Mix up the rules when playing. Sometimes, the offense is allowed only three dribbles to score. Other times, make it unlimited dribbles. While challenging your teammates or another opponent, make it a point to try different defensive strategies when guarding them. This will help you improve on the defensive weaknesses that you have. For instance, don't just sag off of the offensive player and give him or her the jump shot. Don't just force the person to the left all the time just because they are right-handed. Instead, play solid defense up close without fouling. Make the person actually work to get a basket, or you get the defensive stop.

As a player, I loved to play one on one. I strive to work on the weak areas of my game during this time. It also was my goal to learn how to defend players of different sizes and abilities. So, I constantly tried different strategies and techniques to learn what actually worked and what didn't. Understanding your own offensive and defensive strengths and weaknesses must be acknowledged. Overall, one on one competition brings out the best in your opponent if you are giving your best. Don't try to just develop one or two "go to" moves. Strive to have your offensive reaction to be based on the situation that's presented to you by the defense.

Champion's Vision Tip #10

1. Be creative on offense when playing one on one games. By trying different move combinations, it helps you learn to react to situations in a variety of ways.

2. Getting a defensive stop before the offensive player is able to shoot the basketball should be the goal when playing one on one games.

3. Practice shooting under pressure (when the defensive person is guarding you up close) during one on one games. This simulates actual game situations.

4. Think two to three possessions ahead on offense and defense when playing one on one. Visualize yourself performing a successful move and scoring

or getting a defensive stop. Then do it in the real game.

5. Challenge different teammates regardless of size or ability of one-on-one games. Work on improving your strengths and weaknesses while playing at a high level.

A Basketball Wish

As the stars light up the sky on a hot summer night, the sound that's heard causes some to take flight. With unwavering force it goes on and on. Many stare wondering when will it be done. Walk after walk and street after street, the challenge that's given is to not miss a beat. As the night grows old nobody's there. There's a pause in the road, along with a prayer.

It all started with this so, I pass it with a no look dish. This...Yes. This is my basketball wish.

By

David Carl Smith Jr.

Notes

Notes

Notes

Notes

Notes

Notes

Notes

Notes

Notes

Notes

Notes

Notes

www.ingramcontent.com/pod-product-compliance
Lightning Source LLC
Chambersburg PA
CBHW052114070526
44584CB00017B/2480